The Atkins Diet

How To Cut Sugar From Your Diet

By PROSENCE

Copyright 2017 by Prosence - All rights reserved.

This document is geared towards providing exact and reliable information in regards to the topic and issue covered. The publication is sold with the idea that the publisher is not required to render accounting, officially permitted, or otherwise, qualified services. If advice is necessary, legal or professional, a practiced individual in the profession should be ordered.

- From a Declaration of Principles which was accepted and approved equally by a Committee of the American Bar Association and a Committee of Publishers and Associations.

The information provided herein is stated to be truthful and consistent, in that any liability, in terms of inattention or otherwise, by any usage or abuse of any policies, processes, or directions contained within is the solitary and utter responsibility of the recipient reader. Under no circumstances will any legal responsibility or blame be held against the publisher for any reparation, damages, or monetary loss due to the information herein, either directly or indirectly.

Respective authors own all copyrights not held by the publisher.

The information herein is offered for informational purposes solely, and is universal as so. The presentation of the information is without contract or any type of guarantee assurance.

The trademarks that are used are without any consent, and the publication of the trademark is without permission or backing by the trademark owner. All trademarks and brands within this book are for clarifying purposes only and are the owned by the owners themselves, not affiliated with this document.

ABOUT PROSENCE

Our Mission

We are dedicated to guiding, motivating and providing the tools necessary to transform people into the best version of themselves. Our goal is to empower men and women across the globe to realize that physical and mental fitness are not a short-term solution, but a lifetime choice- and to actualize what they have come to understand into a daily routine. We invite you to discover this process for yourself as you join us in the exploration of science-based knowledge that can lead to better health, greater fulfillment and astonishing vitality.

Who is Prosence?

Hi, I'm Antonio Mazzotta - certified Fitness Trainer and health enthusiast, and the founder of Prosence. While I don't think I'll ever turn down mom's homemade pasta and pizza, as an Italian living in Switzerland I've built a life dedicated to health and fitness. Now, I want to share the secrets to my success with you.

I got involved in this industry over 7 years ago, and quickly developed a passion for all things health and fitness. I knew right away that this is what I was born to do and haven't looked back. My days are spent developing new routines, training hard and meeting other fitness-minded and health-conscious individuals. I love working with my clients and coaching about weight training, dieting and healthy lifestyle choices. My number one priority is motivating people to achieve any fitness goal they seek. Whether you're looking to lose weight, get stronger, build cardio and endurance or just maintain overall health and vitality - I'm here to get you to your goals.

My team and I work hard to dispel the health and fitness myths and misinformation clogging the Internet today. We're driven by the desire to offer you a safe and manageable yet powerfully effective path to the best health of your life. Prosence is firmly committed to motivating, inspiring, and educating through the sharing of objective, fact-based health and fitness information that is rooted in science. We give you the tools you need to get in great shape and build a lifetime of good health.

Join us - let's work together to maximize your potential and achieve your optimal self while embracing life to the fullest!

Learn more on our website: www.prosencefitness.com, blog and keep up with the daily education and motivation by liking us on Twitter, Facebook & Instagram @prosencefitness.

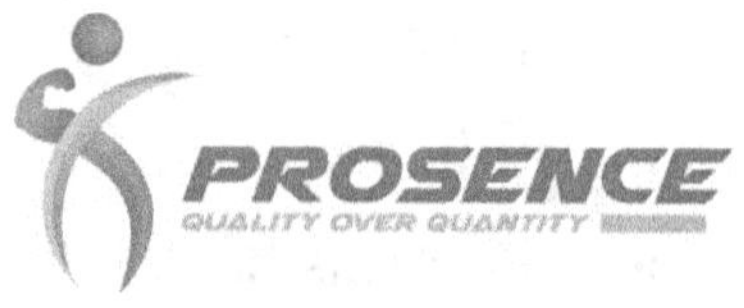

Table of Contents

Introduction

I would like to thank you for purchasing this book "The Atkins Diet: How to cut sugar from your diet."

Wouldn't it be nice if you could improve your overall health by cutting down on your consumption of sugars? Do you want to achieve your weight loss and health goals without having to cut down on your food intake? If yes, then the Atkins diet is meant for you!

The Atkins diet isn't one of the fad diets, and it has been in existence for a while now. Dr. Robert Atkins, a cardiologist, is the creator this popular and successful diet. The objective of this diet is to recognize various food groups that are a perfect match for your metabolism. It might sound entirely different from all the other diets, but it is true. When Dr. Robert Atkins started researching about various diets, he introduced his patients to a low sugar and a low-carb diet. His theory is quite simple; he believed that the human body neither needs sugar nor carbs for survival and he was right.

In this book, you will learn the basics of the Atkins diet, the various benefits it offers, and the different phases of this diet. Not just that, this book also answers multiple FAQs about this brilliant diet and an Atkins-friendly food list that will help you in following the diet. So, why don't we get started?

Chapter 1
About The Atkins Diet

The Atkins diet is a low-carb diet, and the aim of this diet is the consumption of foods that work well with your metabolism for losing weight. The diet works in four phases, and each of these stages assists in weight loss. Dr. Atkins believed that human beings usually ignored specific essential factors when it comes to their eating habits. These factors are the primary cause of unnecessary weight gain. All the refined carbs and processed foods we have are the leading cause of obesity these days.

When you start following the protocols of Atkins diet, you will notice that your body is burning up all the excess fat stored in your body instead of burning glucose for producing energy. The switch in your body's metabolism is ketosis. The insulin level in your body is directly proportional to the concentration of glucose in your bloodstream. A low level of glucose means a low level of insulin. When this happens, ketosis sets in. When your body is in ketosis, it starts utilizing the stored fats.

Usually, your body tends to have a low level of glucose and insulin before eating. Once you consume food, the level of glucose rises and this, in turn, causes the insulin level to increase. When you have lots of carbohydrates, your bloodstream is flooded with glucose. A couple of carbs, known as the "good" carbs don't have a severe effect on your glucose levels. These specific carbohydrates help in the transfer of stored fat from the cells to the bloodstream during ketosis.

Dr. Atkins created a low carb diet that triggers the body's metabolism, and it enables your body to burn more calories than it usually does. During this process, your body also gets rid of all the extra calories that it was storing.

Dr. Atkins coined the term Net Carbs, and it refers to the total carbohydrates consumed minus all the sugar alcohols and fiber. It was observed that the sugar alcohols don't have any effect on your blood sugar levels. Dr. Atkins truly believed that all those carbs with a low glycemic load are best suited. After thorough research, he concluded that the consumption of saturated fats shouldn't be more than 20% of the total calorie intake.

Four phases of the Atkins Diet

Phase 1: Induction

You have to make sure that there's a reduction in your daily calorie intake. Once your body gets acclimatized to this change, you have to ensure that your carbohydrate intake is restricted to only 20 grams per day. The primary source of these carbohydrates should be from vegetables and salads that have low starch content.

Phase 2: Ongoing Weight Loss

You should start including foods that are rich in different nutrients and fiber. These are additional sources of carbs, and you have to increase the carb intake to 25 grams during the first week of phase 2 and then keep increasing the intake by five grams every week until you find that there isn't any weight loss. When you reach this stage, you have to slowly cut down your carb intake by 5 grams until you reach a stage when you start losing weight again.

Phase 3: Pre-maintenance

The third phase of the Atkins diet starts when you are just ten pounds away from the goal you have set. You can shed those last 10 pounds during this stage, and it helps in getting your body fine-tuned to focus on your primary health objective.

Phase 4: Lifetime Maintenance

Atkins isn't a temporary diet, and it is a lifestyle change. You should start introducing different sources of carbohydrates at this stage. Monitor your weight carefully to avoid any weight gain. If you feel that you are gaining weight, then there are two options available to you. You can either reduce your carb intake or start eliminating any new carbs that have you been adding to your diet.

Chapter 2
Benefits Of The Atkins Diet

Weight loss isn't the only benefit of the Atkins diet. The various advantages of following the Atkins diet are discussed in this section. So, read on to learn more.

Epilepsy and related diseases

Approximately 35 studies conducted between 2004 and 2014 show that the Atkins diet can help in reducing epilepsy and other seizure disorders in children and adults alike. These studies proved to be encouraging for children diagnosed with epilepsy, especially those who haven't been responding well to any medication.

GERD

Studies show that any low-carb diet, like the Atkins, can help in easing acid reflux. Foods that are fatty or have a high level of caffeine encourage acid reflux. Atkins diet being a low carb diet has a positive effect on GERD.

Acne

A review that was published in Skin Pharmacology and Physiology, after a lot of research, shows that a low carb diet can help in reducing the breaking out of acne.

Heart diseases

Between the years 2002 and 2014, twenty-one studies were conducted to identify the effect a low-carb diet has on the heart's health. It was found that a diet, like the Atkins, helps in reducing the risk factor of suffering from heart diseases. It also helps in reducing hypertension and the levels of cholesterol and triglycerides too. Not just that, it helps in preventing inflammation of glands and thereby efficiently controls the various triggers of heart diseases.

Cancer

Obesity is a leading factor that increases the risk of certain types of cancer. Therefore, by following a low-carb diet, you can successfully reduce this risk and also maintain your ideal weight.

Polycystic Ovary Syndrome

It is a common problem that affects women in the reproductive age group. It is a problem that's related to obesity, resistance to insulin, and hyperinsulinemia. A low-carb and a low-sugar diet can help in reducing the body's insulin resistance.

Dementia

A high calorific diet is associated with an increase in the risk of damage to the cognitive portion of the brain. All those who have a high-calorie carb and sugar diet are at a higher risk of suffering from dementia. The Atkins diet would make sure that this risk is lowered.

Chapter 3
Change Your Mindset To Lose Weight

Reversing the leadership model

People who want to lose weight fall into two categories typically. The first group includes those who prefer to fight the battle privately and seclude themselves. The second type constitutes the "would-be dieters" consulting and listening to nutritionists, doctors, trainers, or even the infomercial sellers before following a diet. There's nothing wrong with either of the groups, and they could both work.

The problem comes up only when the follower gets tired of following instructions. Once you get tired of following the strict rules, you will feel like giving in to your temptations. The problem lies with the dieters. What is required is a well-balanced program of leading and following. You have to take back some of the control that you have unknowingly passed on to the experts. You shouldn't do something just because your nutritionist asked you to. You should realize that you are following the diet for your own good and not for someone else's sake. You should want to do something for your benefit, and you should believe in the cause.

Let go of the fear

In the world of weight-loss, fear is almost as bad as a chocolate cake. You might fear the weighing scale, the doctor's appointment, shopping for clothes, of taking pictures or of just being embarrassed. You are bound to retreat if you start fearing everything. The feat can be genuine and tough to fight off.

So, this is where the concept of setting goals comes into the picture. You needn't set big goals; it can be a small goal as well. Set goals that are attainable. It could be something as simple as abstaining from eating chocolates or cookies for a week! You should set a physical and a mental challenge for yourself, something that would scare you to make a good choice because choices are the means for attaining that goal. Set a task for yourself and a deadline for accomplishing it. This will give you the motivation required to keep you going.

Crank up the voltage

You should have a positive mindset if you want to lose all those excess kilos you are holding on to. Slow and steady wins the race. The choices that you make over a period will dictate your progress. Change takes time, and it isn't overnight. The same holds true for dieting as well. It is not just about changing your diet; you should throw in some exercise into the mix if you want to reach your weight goal. You will be successful at following a diet only if it doesn't feel like a punishment to you. You should enjoy the experience the way a child would enjoy recess. Indulge in physical activities that excite you. The byproduct of genuinely investing yourself in something is that you will be able to find what you were looking for without any extra effort. If you are serious about following the Atkins diet, then you will have to change your mindset a little. Keep trying new recipes; diet doesn't mean bland food. Keep things interesting, on days when you crave something that you shouldn't eat you can come up with cheat snacks to fulfill your cravings. Don't think of the diet as a punishment, think of it as a means to a healthier life.

Chapter 4
Mistakes To Avoid

The common mistakes that people tend to make while following the Atkins diet are discussed in this section.

Don't count your total carbs

You needn't count the total carbs you consume in a day while following this diet. Instead, you should keep track of your Net Carbs (Total carbs minus the grams of fiber absorbed). You shouldn't forget to include the acceptable condiments like lemon juice and various sugar substitutes while calculating your net carbs. Use your carb allowance wisely and don't use it for consuming foods that are rich in sugar and carbs and low in fiber. Don't skip carbs altogether. Make sure that you are having the minimum requirement of carbohydrates for your body to function normally.

Skipping veggies

You shouldn't skimp on vegetables. Make sure that 75% of your minimum carbohydrate consumption is from vegetables. It means that you should eat at least two cups of cooked greens, and up to 6 cups of leafy vegetables every day.

Not drinking water

You should be drinking at least 8 cups of water daily, and this can increase with the increase in physical activity. As long as your urine is pale or clear, it indicates that you are drinking sufficient water. Two cups can be in the form of coffee or tea, broth or sugar-free drinks. It will be a misguided attempt if you skimp on fluids just to see a lower score on the weighing machine. If you don't drink sufficient water, your body will start retaining water as a precautionary measure.

Avoiding salt

You need to consume a little salt; you shouldn't skip it altogether. You can avoid feeling headaches, weakness and even muscle cramps by having a small amount of salt when your body is transitioning from burning carbohydrates to fat for generating energy. Atkins is a diuretic diet, and therefore you needn't avoid salt. However, you should limit your salt intake if you are suffering from hypertension or if you have been advised to do so by your doctor.

Not eating sufficient protein

You have to consume somewhere between 4 to 6 ounces of protein for each meal, depending on your age, height and gender. Four ounces might be sufficient for a petite woman, but a man might need up to 6 ounces. It doesn't mean that you should consume only protein and skip vegetables, overeat protein or vice versa. Doing this will interfere with your weight loss, and you will also be subjected to severe cravings for carbs.

Being scared of fat

Certain dietary fats are essential for the body to burn the fat and these natural fats are fine when you are mindful of your carb intake. You should always accompany a snack of carbohydrates with either fat or protein.

Consuming hidden carbs

Read the labels on packaged food items carefully. Just because the package says low calorie, don't assume that it means low carb as well. Make sure that you are using full-fat versions of mayonnaise, salad dressings, and related products. The low-fat versions tend to mix in additional sugar to replace the flavor that's added by oil.

Neglecting to record your progress

You shouldn't forget to register your progress. Maintain a journal for making all your weekly entries regarding your weight and measurements. You can also include a food journal to keep track of the carbs you are consuming. Tracking your progress will help you make the necessary changes to your diet so that it would suit your metabolism well.

Chapter 5
Atkins Food List

Foods to avoid

- Processed foods that contain sugar, like soft drinks, cakes, chocolates, ice cream and so on.

- All grains like wheat, rye, rice, barley, and so on.

- Vegetable oils like corn oil, canola oil, soybean oil and a few others as well.

- Food items that contain trans-fat or hydrogenated oils should be avoided.

- So-called "diet" and "low-fat" food products.

- Skip high carb vegetables like potatoes, carrots, turnips, etc. during the induction phase.

- During induction avoid high carb fruits like banana, grapes, oranges, and pears

- You should also avoid all legumes during the induction phase.

Foods that you should eat

- Include different meats like lamb, chicken, beef, pork, bacon and turkey.

- Fatty fish like salmon, trout, sardines and other seafood as well.

- Consume eggs because they are rich in Omega 3

- All low-carb vegetables should be included like kale, spinach, broccoli, bell peppers and so on.

- Full-fat dairy products like milk, butter, cream, cheese, and yogurt.

- Nuts and seeds like almonds, cashews, walnuts, sunflower seeds, pumpkin seeds and so on.

- Include healthy fats like olive oil, coconut oil, avocados, etc.

Grocery list

Whenever you go for your weekly grocery shopping, you don't have to opt for organic produce. Whenever possible, opt for it. Stick to your grocery list and don't buy any sorts of processed or packaged foods.

- Meats such as beef, chicken, lamb, pork, and bacon.

- Fatty fish like salmon, trout, mackerel and so on.

- Include seafood like prawns and other shellfish.

- Eggs.

- Full-fat dairy products like cream, butter, cheese, milk and yogurt.

- Vegetables such as spinach, lettuce, kale, broccoli, bell peppers, cauliflower, cabbage, asparagus, onions, Brussels sprouts and so on.

- Fruits like apples, pears, oranges, watermelon, and muskmelon.

- Berries like strawberries, blueberries, raspberries, etc.

- Nuts like cashew nuts, almonds, macadamia, hazelnuts, pistachios, etc.

- Olives.

- Extra virgin olive oil, coconut oil or avocado oil.

- Avocados.

- Dark chocolate comes in handy when you crave something sweet.

- Various condiments like pepper, sea salt, garlic, chili powder, turmeric, coriander, parsley, etc.

It will be helpful if you can clear your pantry of all undesirable and unhealthy foods like ice creams, cookies, breakfast cereals, bread, packaged juices and drinks, sugar, etc.

The Atkins diet is about eating healthy and wholesome foods that are good for you. You will need to enjoy what you are eating, and it shouldn't feel like a punishment for you. You don't really have to stock up on expensive pre-cooked meals or anything of that sort. You can eat the regular everyday ingredients, and the only change that you will be making to your diet is to avoid consuming carbs and sugar. That's all that there is to the Atkins diet. You needn't even worry when you are going out for a meal or traveling.

Chapter 6
Atkins FAQs

The Atkins diet is all about eating foods that are well suited for your body metabolism. In the previous chapter, you have learned about all such foods that you can and cannot consume. Keep the list in mind whenever you are picking up groceries. You should learn about the foods that will help you shed weight and start cutting down on empty carbs by avoiding sugar. Learn to read labels thoroughly and carefully. Understand the ingredients and read the nutritional facts before you purchase a food product.

Can I customize the diet?

The diet plan that you select would depend on the weight that you are trying to lose. The two primary variations of the Atkins diet are the Atkins 20 and the Atkins 40. In Atkins 20 you can consume up to 20 grams of Net Carbs, and in Atkins 40 you can consume 40 grams of Net Carbs on a daily basis. Apart from this, there are various other food products you can eat, and you should make sure that you are following the diet plan that you have selected.

How to keep track of what I eat?

It is essential that you keep track of the number of carbs that you are consuming while on the Atkins diet. Before you get started with keeping track of all that you are eating, you will first need to understand the concept of Net Carbs. Net Carbs is different from Total Carbs. You can also make use of various online carb counters for counting all the carbs you are consuming on a daily basis. Make sure that you are sticking to the list of Atkins-friendly foods. It is essential that you are keeping track of your progress. Improvement doesn't just mean the weight that you have lost but also the manner in which you have improved your health. Once every week, you should weigh yourself and note down your measurements as well. You should maintain a food journal as well for keeping track of all that you have been consuming through the day. Record your exercising schedule and any other activity that you think would influence your diet.

Should I worry about the portion size?

When you are following the Atkins diet, you needn't have to worry about your calorie consumption. Just make sure that you are allowing your common sense to guide you through the diet. Consumption of calories is essential for your wellbeing, but you shouldn't overdo it. If you consume more calories than what your body is capable of burning, then it will slow down the process of weight loss. But if you cut down on your calorie intake drastically, then it will slow down your metabolism and will hinder weight loss as well.

Will I be starving myself?

When you are on the Atkins diet, make sure that you keep eating at regular intervals. You can consume five or six small meals throughout the day. Stick to the foods that are mentioned in this book and avoid the ones you shouldn't. As long as you are eating what you are allowed to eat, and the portions are regular sized, then you needn't worry about your calorie intake. If you starve yourself, your blood sugar levels will drop, and it would lead to undesirable consequences that are entirely avoidable. If you want to be able to control your appetite and ensure that your energy levels are high, then you really shouldn't starve yourself.

Should I include protein in all my meals?

You will have to include protein in one form or the other in all your meals. Depending on your age and gender you should consume 4 to 6 ounces of protein on a daily basis. When on the Atkins diet, you can choose from a wide range of proteins, depending on what you fancy. You can consume eggs, fatty meats or even lean meat, seafood and shellfish, and any other form of poultry as well. If you like red meat, then you can opt for a fancy marbled cut of beef. Ensure that whatever protein you have chosen, you are cooking it with plenty of olive oil and also that the salads have sufficient dressing as well.

Is naturally fatty food good for me?

Fatty food tastes so much better than non-greasy food. Greasy food also tends to fill you up quicker than non-fatty food or lean food. Dietary fat is essential when on the Atkins diet. It is necessary for maintaining your overall health. However, dietary fat doesn't mean trans-fat; so, stay away from it. Dietary fat is essential for your metabolic functions and skipping fats altogether is a terrible and dangerous idea. Consuming olive oil, full-fat dairy products and even fat cuts of meats will provide you the much-needed dietary fats.

Can I include sugar?

All the soft drinks and other junk food tend to contain a lot of added sugar and these need to be avoided at all costs. All processed foods include added sugars that are high in calories and low in nutrients. You could opt for non-caloric sweeteners for sweetening your drinks like Stevia or Sucralose. You should ensure that your daily Net Carbs doesn't exceed 3 grams for all these non-caloric sweeteners. As a rule of thumb, stay away from all packaged foods or foods that look like they are manufactured in a factory.

Am I allowed to eat all vegetables?

You shouldn't skip or cut down on veggies. Vegetables are essential for you, and they provide the necessary fiber and nutrients that your body needs. You will have to make sure that at least 75% of your daily carbohydrate intake comes from vegetables. It means that you must include 5-6 servings of vegetables throughout the day. Make sure that you are getting sufficient fiber every day. Fiber helps in controlling the levels of blood sugar in the body and makes you feel fuller for longer, thereby assisting in maintaining your weight.

How much water should I be drinking?

You should keep yourself hydrated to make sure that the electrolyte composition of your body isn't disturbed. You need to drink eight glasses of water at least and depending on the level of activity that you indulge in; you can drink more water. You can consume a healthy broth or non-caffeinated drinks. Green tea is a good option. If you don't drink sufficient water, it will lead to water retentions. When your body is well hydrated, you can get rid of the water weight.

What about daily supplements?

When you are on a diet, you should take a few vitamin and nutrient supplements. It is not just about skipping carbohydrates, but it is about consuming the right food for your body. Your body needs specific nutrients, and if your daily diet doesn't provide those nutrients, it can lead to complications. You should consult your nutritionist or your doctor before you decide to take any supplements. The regular supplements recommended include supplements of iron, calcium, mineral, potassium, and omega-3 and magnesium.

Can I include some physical activity as well?

Your body metabolism will improve if you indulge in some physical activity. Atkins diet is not just a diet but also a lifestyle choice. If you want to keep the weight that you have lost at bay, then the physical activity is as significant as following the diet. You needn't necessarily have to go to the gym to exercise; you can go for swimming, brisk walking, and yoga, dancing, Zumba, or you can even play an outdoor game like basketball or tennis. You will not only start burning calories rapidly but will also begin building muscle.

What about additional support?

Your family and friends would be your support system. Talk to them about the diet and the dietary restrictions that you have. Get them to understand what you should and shouldn't be doing for your own wellbeing. When the going gets tough, and at times you might also feel like quitting, your family and friends will keep you motivated to keep going.

Should I plan in advance?

If you are committed to following this diet, then it is essential that you plan for all your meals. Your kitchen should be stocked up with all the necessary foods that you can consume while on the Atkins diet. If you don't have the required ingredients on hand when you are hungry, it is very likely that you will fall back into your old habits. One thing that you can do is cook in batches and freeze it. Whenever you have some spare time, you can plan and prep for the next few meals.

Conclusion

I would like to thank you once again for purchasing this book. I hope it proved to be an informative read.

In this book, you were provided with all the information that you would need for getting started with the Atkins diet. The Atkins diet is so much more than a diet; it is a lifestyle change that will help in improving your overall health by working alongside your body metabolism. There are different benefits this diet offers, and it isn't restricted to just weight loss. You can successfully lose weight, maintain the weight loss, and improve your immunity as well. The Atkins diet is a low sugar and a low-carb diet that is quite easy to follow. The grocery list provided in this book will help you in gathering all the necessary supplies so that you can cook healthy and nutritious food easily. Not just that, the simple tricks that are discussed will make it easy to follow the diet. All that's left for you to do is to get started with this diet. It isn't difficult, and a little extra effort goes a long way. The Atkins diet will work wonders for you, and you will be able to see a positive change in your body. So, get going and all the best!

If you enjoyed this book then I'd like to ask you for a favor. Will you be kind enough to leave a review for this book on Amazon? It would be greatly appreciated!

Don't forget to follow us on Twitter, Facebook & Instagram and visit our website www.prosencefitness.com to get empowered, educated and inspired to become the best version of yourself in life! You deserve it.

Resources

https://www.atkins.com/how-it-works/faqs/product-faq

https://googleweblight.com/i?u=https://www.atkins.com/how-it-works/atkins-blogs/colette-heimowitz/benefits-of-atkins-diet-beyond-weight-loss&grqid=a45w_qGw&hl=en-IN

https://www.healthline.com/nutrition/atkins-diet-101

http://googleweblight.com/i?u=http://diet.lovetoknow.com/wiki/Atkins_Diet_Food_List&grqid=KiggUJWJ&hl=en-IN